Mediterranean Savory Recipes

50 Tasty & Quick Recipes to Cook Your Daily Mediterranean Meals

Carmen Berlanti

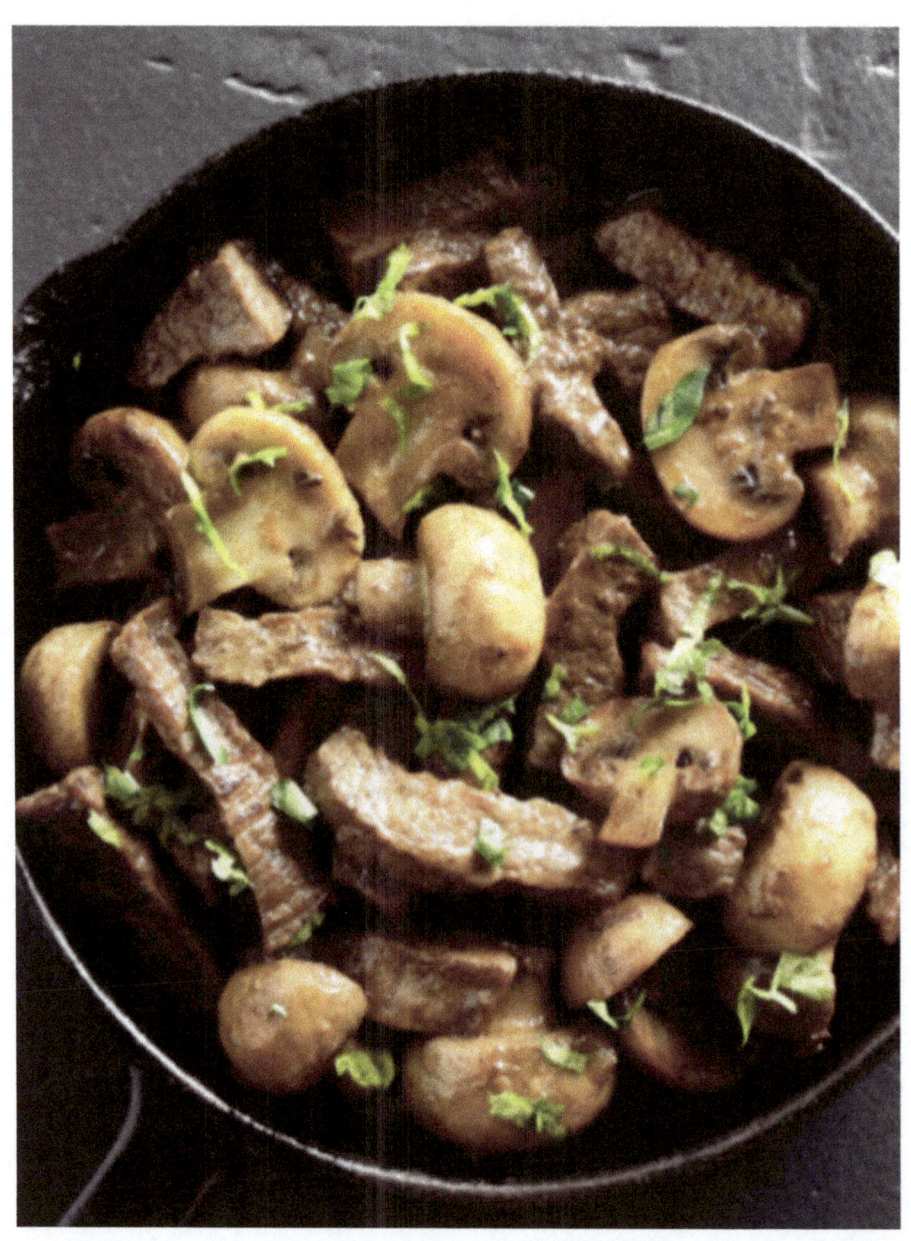

© Copyright 2021 - All rights reserved.

The content contained within this book may not be reproduced, duplicated or transmitted without direct written permission from the author or the publisher.
Under no circumstances will any blame or legal responsibility be held against the publisher, or author, for any damages, reparation, or monetary loss due to the information contained within this book. Either directly or indirectly.

Legal Notice:
This book is copyright protected. This book is only for personal use. You cannot amend, distribute, sell, use, quote or paraphrase any part, or the content within this book, without the consent of the author or publisher.

Disclaimer Notice:
Please note the information contained within this document is for educational and entertainment purposes only. All effort has been executed to present accurate, up to date, and reliable, complete information. No warranties of any kind are declared or implied. Readers acknowledge that the author is not engaging in the rendering of legal, financial, medical or professional advice. The content within this book has been derived from various sources. Please consult a licensed professional before attempting any techniques outlined in this book.

By reading this document, the reader agrees that under no circumstances is the author responsible for any losses, direct or indirect, which are incurred as a result of the use of information contained within this document, including, but not limited to, — errors, omissions, or inaccuracies.

Table of Contents

Roasted Red Pepper Hummus 7

Roasted Rosemary Olives 10

Spiced Maple Nuts 12

Greek Turkey Burger 15

Za'atar Chicken Tenders 18

Yogurt-Marinated Chicken Kebabs 20

Honey Ricotta with Espresso and Chocolate Chips 23

Figs with Mascarpone and Honey 25

Pistachio-Stuffed Dates 27

Yogurt Tahini Dressing 29

Portable Packed Picnic Pieces 32

Naturally Nutty & Buttery Banana Bowl 34

Cannellini Beans with Rosemary and Garlic Aioli 36

Ful Medames 38

Fresh Sauce Pasta 40

Penne in Tomato and Caper Sauce 42

Tahini Sauce 44

Basil Pesto 46

Barley Porridge 48

Spiced Almond Pancakes 50

Artichoke Frittata 52

Fennel Wild Rice 56

Brussels Sprouts with Pistachios 58

Roasted Parmesan Broccoli 60

Mashed Celeriac 62

Herbed Yogurt Dip 64

Southwest Pizza 66

Spinach Chicken Pizza 68

Linguine with Cherry Tomatoes	70
Linguine with Tomato Clam Sauce	72
Angel Hair with Asparagus-Kale Pesto	74
Cucumber Hummus Sandwiches	76
Blackberries Caprese Skewers	77
Tomato-Basil Skewers	78
Fig and Ricotta Toast	80
Date Wraps	82
Easy Stuffed Peppers	83
Buttery Carrot Sticks	85
Cajun Walnuts and Olives Bowls	87
Mango Salsa	89
Crisp Spiced Cauliflower with Feta Cheese	91
Spring Peas and Beans with Zesty Thyme Yogurt Sauce	93
Breakfast Pita	96
Beef with Pesto Sandwich	98
Classic Steak Panini	100
Grilled Sandwich with Goat Cheese	102
Fried Green Tomatoes	105
One-of-a-Kind Veggie Slaw	107
Ratatouille Grilled Style	109

Roasted Red Pepper Hummus

Difficulty Level: 1/5

Preparation time: *15 minutes*

Cooking time: *0 minutes*

Servings: *2 cups*

Ingredients:

1 (15-ounce) can low-sodium chickpeas, drained and rinsed

3 ounces jarred roasted red bell peppers, drained

3 tablespoons tahini

3 tablespoons lemon juice

1 garlic clove, peeled

¾ teaspoon kosher salt

¼ teaspoon freshly ground black pepper

3 tablespoons extra-virgin olive oil

¼ teaspoon cayenne pepper (optional)

Fresh herbs, chopped, for garnish (optional)

Directions:

In a food processor, add the chickpeas, red bell peppers, tahini, lemon juice, garlic, salt, and black pepper. Pulse 5 to 7 times. Add the olive oil and process until smooth. Add the cayenne pepper and garnish with chopped herbs, if desired.

Nutrition:

Per serving (1/4 cup)

Calories: 130

Total fat: 8g

Saturated fat: 1g

Cholesterol: 0mg

Sodium: 150mg

Potassium: 125mg

Total Carbohydrates: 11g

Fiber: 2g

Sugars: 1g

Protein: 4g

Magnesium: 20mg

Calcium: 48mg

Roasted Rosemary Olives

Difficulty Level: 2/5

Preparation time: *5 minutes*

Cooking time: *25 minutes*

Servings: *4*

Ingredients:

1 cup mixed variety olives, pitted and rinsed

2 tablespoons lemon juice

1 tablespoon extra-virgin olive oil

6 garlic cloves, peeled

4 rosemary sprigs

Directions:

Preheat the oven to 400°F. Line the baking sheet with parchment paper or foil.

Combine the olives, lemon juice, olive oil, and garlic in a medium bowl and mix together. Spread in a single layer on the prepared baking sheet. Sprinkle on the rosemary. Roast for 25 minutes, tossing halfway through.

Remove the rosemary leaves from the stem and place in a serving bowl. Add the olives and mix before serving.

Nutrition:

Per serving

Calories: 100

Total fat: 9g

Saturated fat: 1g

Cholesterol: 0mg

Sodium: 260mg

Potassium: 31mg

Total Carbohydrates: 4g

Fiber: 0g

Sugars: 0g

Protein: 0g

Magnesium: 3mg

Calcium: 11mg

Spiced Maple Nuts

Difficulty Level: 2/5

Preparation time: *5 minutes*

Cooking time: *10 minutes*

Servings: *2 cups*

Ingredients:

2 cups raw walnuts or pecans (or a mix of nuts)

1 teaspoon extra-virgin olive oil

1 teaspoon ground sumac

½ teaspoon pure maple syrup

¼ teaspoon kosher salt

¼ teaspoon ground ginger

2 to 4 rosemary sprigs

Directions:

Preheat the oven to 350°F. Line a baking sheet with parchment paper or foil.

In a large bowl, combine the nuts, olive oil, sumac, maple syrup, salt, and ginger; mix together. Spread in a single layer on the prepared baking sheet. Add the rosemary. Roast for 8 to 10 minutes, or until golden and fragrant.

Remove the rosemary leaves from the stems and place in a serving bowl. Add the nuts and toss to combine before serving.

Nutrition:

Per serving (1/4 cup)

Calories: 175

Total fat: 18g

Saturated fat: 2g

Cholesterol: 0mg

Sodium: 35mg

Potassium: 110mg

Total Carbohydrates: 4g

Fiber: 2g

Sugars: 1g

Protein: 3g

Magnesium: 35mg

Calcium: 23mg

Greek Turkey Burger

Difficulty Level: 2/5

Preparation time: *10 minutes*

Cooking time: *10 minutes*

Servings: *4*

Ingredients:

1 pound ground turkey

1 medium zucchini, grated

¼ cup whole-wheat bread crumbs

¼ cup red onion, minced

¼ cup crumbled feta cheese

1 large egg, beaten

1 garlic clove, minced

1 tablespoon fresh oregano, chopped

1 teaspoon kosher salt

¼ teaspoon freshly ground black pepper

1 tablespoon extra-virgin olive oil

Directions:

In a large bowl, combine the turkey, zucchini, bread crumbs, onion, feta cheese, egg, garlic, oregano, salt, and black pepper, and mix well. Shape into 4 equal patties.

Heat the olive oil in a large nonstick grill pan or skillet over medium-high heat. Add the burgers to the pan and reduce the heat to medium. Cook on one side for 5 minutes, then flip and cook the other side for 5 minutes more.

SUBSTITUTION TIP: Any summer squash can be used in this recipe, so feel free to swap out the zucchini for yellow squash or pattypan squash.

Nutrition:

Per serving

Calories: 285

Total fat: 16g

Saturated fat: 5g

Cholesterol: 139mg

Sodium: 465mg

Potassium: 415mg

Total Carbohydrates: 9g

Fiber: 2g

Sugars: 2g

Protein: 26g

Magnesium: 40mg

Calcium: 90mg

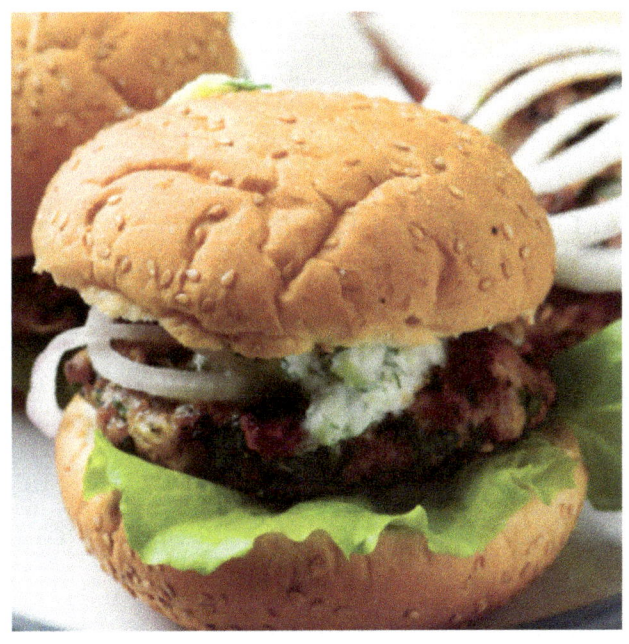

Za'atar Chicken Tenders

Difficulty Level: 2/5

Preparation time: *5 minutes*

Cooking time: *15 minutes*

Servings: *4*

Ingredients:

Olive oil cooking spray

1 pound chicken tenders

1½ tablespoons za'atar

½ teaspoon kosher salt

¼ teaspoon freshly ground black pepper

Directions:

Preheat the oven to 450°F. Line a baking sheet with parchment paper or foil and lightly spray with olive oil cooking spray.

In a large bowl, combine the chicken, za'atar, salt, and black pepper. Mix together well, covering the chicken tenders fully. Arrange in a single layer on the baking sheet and bake for 15 minutes, turning the chicken over once halfway through the cooking time.

Nutrition:

Per serving

Calories: 145

Total fat: 4g

Saturated fat: 1g

Cholesterol: 83mg

Sodium: 190mg

Potassium: 390mg

Total Carbohydrates: 0g

Fiber: 0g

Sugars: 0g

Protein: 26g

Magnesium: 37mg

Calcium: 13mg

Yogurt-Marinated Chicken Kebabs

Difficulty Level: 2/5

Preparation time: 10 *minutes*

Cooking time: *20 minutes*

Servings: *4*

Ingredients:

½ cup plain Greek yogurt

1 tablespoon lemon juice

½ teaspoon ground cumin

½ teaspoon ground coriander

½ teaspoon kosher salt

¼ teaspoon cayenne pepper

1½ pound skinless, boneless chicken breast, cut into 1-inch cubes

Directions:

In a large bowl or zip-top bag, combine the yogurt, lemon juice, cumin, coriander, salt, and cayenne pepper. Mix together thoroughly and then add the chicken. Marinate for at least 30 minutes, and up to overnight in the refrigerator.

Preheat the oven to 425°F. Line a baking sheet with parchment paper or foil. Remove the chicken from the marinade and thread it on 4 bamboo or metal skewers.

Bake for 20 minutes, turning the chicken over once halfway through the cooking time.

Nutrition:

Per serving

Calories: 170

Total fat: 4g

Saturated fat: 1g

Cholesterol: 92mg

Sodium: 390mg

Potassium: 515mg

Total Carbohydrates: 1g

Fiber: 0g

Sugars: 1g

Protein: 31g

Magnesium: 40mg

Calcium: 35mg

Honey Ricotta with Espresso and Chocolate Chips

Difficulty Level: 1/5

Preparation time: *5 minutes*

Cooking time: *0 minutes*

Servings: *2*

Ingredients:

8 ounces ricotta cheese

2 tablespoons honey

2 tablespoons espresso, chilled or room temperature

1 teaspoon dark chocolate chips or chocolate shavings

Directions:

In a medium bowl, whip together the ricotta cheese and honey until light and smooth, 4 to 5 minutes.

Spoon the ricotta cheese–honey mixture evenly into 2 dessert bowls. Drizzle 1 tablespoon espresso into each dish and sprinkle with chocolate chips or shavings.

SUBSTITUTION TIP: Regular or decaf black coffee can be used in place of the espresso.

Nutrition:

Per serving

Calories: 235

Total fat: 10g

Saturated fat: 6g

Cholesterol: 35mg

Sodium: 115mg

Potassium: 170mg

Total Carbohydrates: 25g

Fiber: 0g

Sugars: 19g

Protein: 13g

Magnesium: 30mg

Calcium: 310mg

Figs with Mascarpone and Honey

Difficulty Level: 2/5

Preparation time: *5 minutes*

Cooking time: *5 minutes*

Servings: *4*

Ingredients:

⅓ cup walnuts, chopped

8 fresh figs, halved

¼ cup mascarpone cheese

1 tablespoon honey

¼ teaspoon flaked sea salt

Directions:

In a skillet over medium heat, toast the walnuts, stirring often, 3 to 5 minutes.

Arrange the figs cut-side up on a plate or platter. Using your finger, make a small depression in the cut side of each fig and fill with mascarpone cheese. Sprinkle with a bit of the walnuts, drizzle with the honey, and add a tiny pinch of sea salt.

Nutrition:

Per serving

Calories: 200

Total fat: 13g

Saturated fat: 4g

Cholesterol: 18mg

Sodium: 105mg

Potassium: 230mg

Total Carbohydrates: 24g

Fiber: 3g

Sugars: 18g

Protein: 3g

Magnesium: 30mg

Calcium: 53mg

Pistachio-Stuffed Dates

Difficulty Level: 1/5

Preparation time: 10 *minutes*

Cooking time: *0 minutes*

Servings: *4*

Ingredients:

½ cup unsalted pistachios, shelled

¼ teaspoon kosher salt

8 Medjool dates, pitted

Directions:

In a food processor, add the pistachios and salt. Process until combined to a chunky nut butter, 3 to 5 minutes.

Split open the dates and spoon the pistachio nut butter into each half.

Nutrition:

Per serving

Calories: 220

Total fat: 7g

Saturated fat: 1g

Cholesterol: 0mg

Sodium: 70mg

Potassium: 490mg

Total Carbohydrates: 41g

Fiber: 5g

Sugars: 33g

Protein: 4g

Magnesium: 43mg

Calcium: 47mg

Yogurt Tahini Dressing

Difficulty Level: *1/5*

Preparation time: *5 minutes*

Cooking time: *0 minutes*

Servings: *1 cup*

Ingredients:

½ cup plain Greek yogurt

⅓ cup tahini

¼ cup freshly squeezed orange juice

½ teaspoon kosher salt

Directions:

In a medium bowl, whisk together the yogurt, tahini, orange juice, and salt until smooth. Place in the refrigerator until ready to serve. Store leftovers in an airtight container in the refrigerator for up to 5 days.

Nutrition:

Per serving (2 tablespoons)

Calories: 70

Total fat: 2g

Saturated fat: 1g

Cholesterol: 0mg

Sodium: 80mg

Potassium: 85mg

Total Carbohydrates: 4g

Fiber: 1g

Sugars: 1g

Protein: 4g

Magnesium: 12mg

Calcium: 66mg

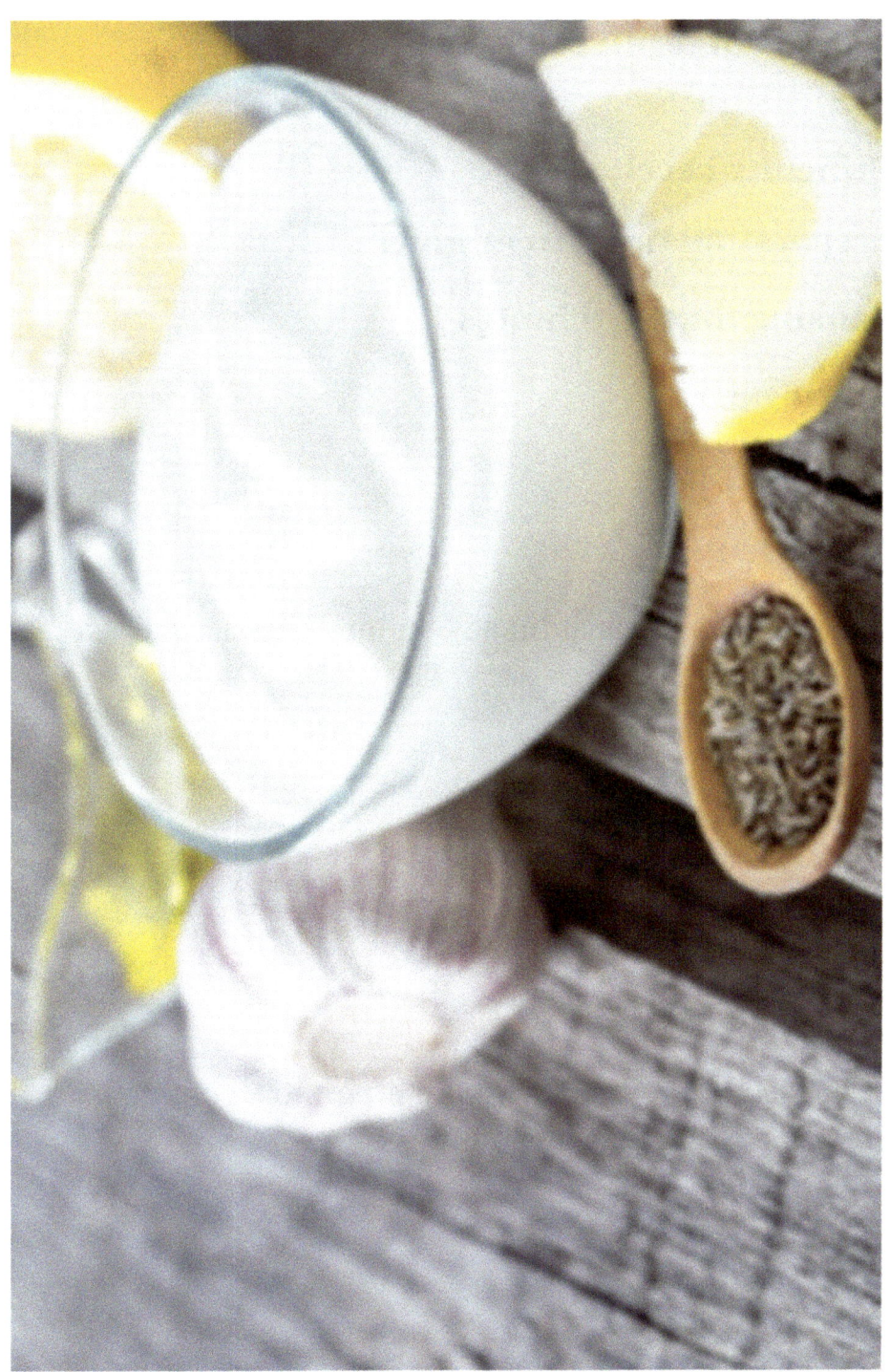

Portable Packed Picnic Pieces

Difficulty Level: 1/5

Preparation time: 10 minutes

Cooking time: 0 minutes

Servings: 1

Ingredients:

1-slice of whole-wheat bread, cut into bite-size pieces

10-pcs cherry tomatoes

¼-oz. aged cheese, sliced

6-pcs oil-cured olives

Directions:

Pack each of the ingredients in a portable container to serve you while snacking on the go.

Nutrition:

Calories: 197

Total Fats: 9g

Fiber: 4g

Carbohydrates: 22g

Protein: 7g

Naturally Nutty & Buttery Banana Bowl

Difficulty Level: 1/5

Preparation time: minutes

Cooking time: 0 minutes

Servings: 4

Ingredients:

4-cups vanilla Greek yogurt

2-pcs medium-sized bananas, sliced

¼-cup creamy and natural peanut butter

1-tsp ground nutmeg

¼-cup flaxseed meal

Directions:

Divide the yogurt equally between four serving bowls. Top each yogurt bowl with the banana slices.

Place the peanut butter in a microwave-safe bowl. Melt the peanut butter in your microwave for 40 seconds. Drizzle one tablespoon of the melted peanut butter over the bananas for each bowl.

To serve, sprinkle over with the ground nutmeg and flax-seed meal.

Nutrition:

Calories: 370

Total Fats: 10.6g

Fiber: 4.7g

Carbohydrates: 47.7g

Protein: 22.7g

Cannellini Beans with Rosemary and Garlic Aioli

Difficulty Level: 2/5

Preparation time: 10 minutes

Cooking time: 10 minutes

Servings: 4

Ingredients:

4 cups cooked cannellini beans (see tip)

4 cups water

½ teaspoon salt

3 tablespoons olive oil

2 tablespoons chopped fresh rosemary

½ cup Garlic Aioli

¼ teaspoon freshly ground black pepper

Directions:

In a medium saucepan over medium heat, combine the cannellini beans, water, and salt. Bring to a boil. Cook for 5 minutes. Drain.

In a skillet over medium heat, heat the olive oil.

Add the beans. Stir in the rosemary and aioli. Reduce the heat to medium-low and cook, stirring, just to heat through. Season with pepper and serve.

Nutrition:

Calories: 545

Total Fats: 36g

Saturated Fat: 6g

Fiber: 14g

Carbohydrates: 42g

Protein: 15g

Sodium: 448mg

Ful Medames

Difficulty Level: 2/5

Preparation time: 15 minutes

Cooking time: 15 minutes

Servings: 6

Ingredients:

1 (15-ounce) can fava beans, undrained

4 garlic cloves, minced

1 tablespoon ground cumin

⅛ teaspoon salt

⅛ teaspoon freshly ground black pepper

½ cup freshly squeezed lemon juice

¼ cup olive oil

1 sweet onion, chopped, divided

2 ripe tomatoes, diced, divided

2 cups finely chopped fresh parsley, divided

Directions:

In a medium saucepan over medium heat, combine the fava beans with their liquid, garlic, cumin, salt, and pepper. Bring to a boil.

Using a potato masher or fork, partially mash the fava beans. Continue to cook over medium heat for 10 minutes more.

Stir in the lemon juice, olive oil, and half each of the onion, tomatoes, and parsley. Taste and season with more salt and pepper, as needed. Remove from the heat.

Spoon the bean mixture into a serving dish and top while hot with the remaining onion, tomatoes, and parsley.

Nutrition:

Calories: 183

Total Fats: 9g

Saturated Fat: 2g

Fiber: 6g

Carbohydrates: 20g

Protein: 15g

Sodium: 74mg

Fresh Sauce Pasta

Difficulty Level: 2/5

Preparation time: 15 minutes

Cooking time: 15 minutes

Servings: 4

Ingredients:

⅛ teaspoon salt, plus more for cooking the pasta

1 pound penne pasta

¼ cup olive oil

1 garlic clove, crushed

3 cups chopped scallions, white and green parts

3 tomatoes, diced

2 tablespoons chopped fresh basil

⅛ teaspoon freshly ground black pepper

Freshly grated Parmesan cheese, for serving

Directions:

Bring a large pot of salted water to a boil over high heat. Drop in the pasta, stir, and return the water to a boil. Boil the pasta for about 6 minutes or until al dente.

A couple minutes before the pasta is completely cooked, in a medium saucepan over medium heat, heat the olive oil.

Add the garlic and cook for 30 seconds.

Stir in the scallions and tomatoes. Cover the pan and cook for 2 to 3 minutes.

Drain the pasta and add it to the vegetables. Stir in the basil and season with the salt and pepper. Top with the Parmesan cheese.

Nutrition:

Calories: 477

Total Fats: 16g

Saturated Fat: 2g

Fiber: 3g

Carbohydrates: 72g

Protein: 15g

Sodium: 120mg

Penne in Tomato and Caper Sauce

Difficulty Level: 2/5

Preparation time: 10 minutes

Cooking time: 15 minutes

Servings: 4

Ingredients:

2 tablespoons olive oil

2 garlic cloves, minced

1 cup sliced cherry tomatoes

2 cups Basic Tomato Basil Sauce, or store-bought

1 cup capers, drained and rinsed

Salt

4 cups penne pasta

Directions:

Set a large pot of salted water over high heat to boil.

In a medium saucepan over medium heat, heat the olive oil. Add the garlic and cook for 30 seconds. Add the cherry tomatoes and cook for 2 to 3 minutes.

Pour in the tomato sauce and bring the mixture to a boil. Stir in the capers and turn off the heat.

Once boiling add the pasta to the pot of water and cook for about 7 minutes until al dente.

Drain the pasta and stir it into the sauce. Toss gently and cook over medium heat for 1 minute or until warmed through.

Nutrition:

Calories: 329

Total Fats: 8g

Saturated Fat: 1g

Fiber: 6g

Carbohydrates: 55g

Protein: 10g

Sodium: 612mg

Tahini Sauce

Difficulty Level: 1/5

Preparation time: 15 minutes

Cooking time: 0 minutes

Servings: 2 cups

Ingredients:

3 garlic cloves, minced or mashed into a paste

½ cup tahini

½ cup freshly squeezed lemon juice

1 cup water

¼ teaspoon ground cumin

⅛ teaspoon salt

4 cups penne pasta

Directions:

In a small bowl, whisk the garlic, tahini, lemon juice, water, cumin, and salt until it develops into a smooth paste. Refrigerate in an airtight container for up to 1 month.

Nutrition:

Per serving (1tablespoon)

Calories: 47

Total Fats: 4g

Saturated Fat: 1g

Fiber: 1g

Carbohydrates: 2g

Protein: 1g

Sodium: 30mg

Basil Pesto

Difficulty Level: 2/5

Preparation time: 15 minutes
Cooking time: 0 minutes
Servings: 1 cup

Ingredients:

2 cups packed chopped fresh basil

3 garlic cloves, peeled

¼ cup pine nuts

½ cup olive oil

½ teaspoon salt

½ cup freshly grated Parmesan cheese

Directions:

1. In a food processor or blender, combine the basil, garlic, and pine nuts. Pulse until coarsely chopped.

Add the olive oil, salt, and Parmesan cheese. Process for 5 minutes until you have a smooth paste.

Refrigerate in an airtight container for up to 3 weeks, or freeze for up to 1 month

Nutrition:

Per serving (1tablespoon)

Calories: 81

Total Fats: 9g

Saturated Fat: 2g

Fiber: 0g

Carbohydrates: 1g

Protein: 2g

Sodium: 91mg

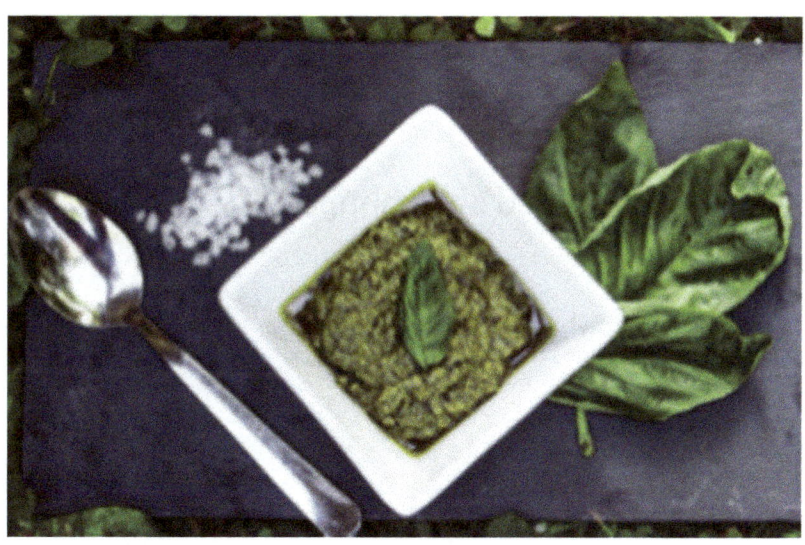

Barley Porridge

Difficulty Level: 2/5

Preparation time: 25 minutes

Cooking time: 5 minutes

Servings: 4

Ingredients:

1 cup barley

1 cup wheat berries

2 cups unsweetened almond milk, plus more for serving

2 cups water

½ cup blueberries

½ cup pomegranate seeds

½ cup hazelnuts, toasted and chopped

¼ cup honey

Directions:

In a medium saucepan over medium-high heat, place the barley, wheat berries, almond milk, and water. Bring to a boil, reduce the heat to low, and simmer for about 25 minutes, stirring frequently until the grains are very tender.

Top each serving with almond milk, 2 tablespoons of blueberries, 2 tablespoons of pomegranate seeds, 2 tablespoons of hazelnuts, and 1 tablespoon of honey.

Nutrition:

Calories: 354;

Total Fat: 8g;

Saturated Fat: 1g;

Carbohydrates: 63g;

Fiber: 10g;

Protein: 11g

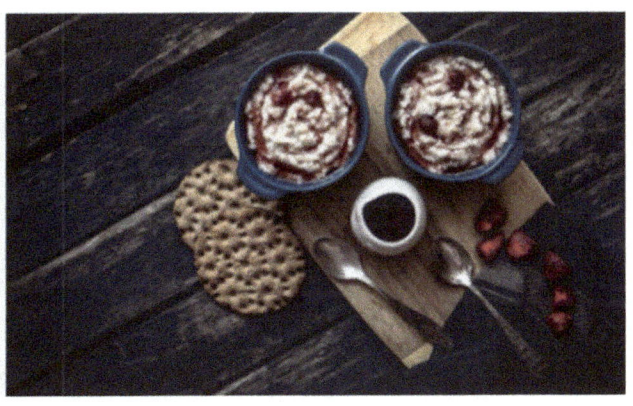

Spiced Almond Pancakes

Difficulty Level: 2/5

Preparation time: 10 minutes

Cooking time: 20 minutes

Servings: 6

Ingredients:

1 pound chicken breasts, cut into medium chunks

12 ounces zucchini, sliced

2 tablespoons olive oil

2 garlic cloves, minced

2 tablespoons parmesan, grated

1 tablespoon parsley, chopped

Salt and black pepper to taste

Directions:

In a large bowl, whisk the almond milk, coconut oil, eggs, and honey until blended.

In a medium bowl, sift together the whole-wheat flour, almond flour, baking powder, baking soda, sea salt, and cinnamon until well mixed.

Add the flour mixture to the milk mixture and whisk until just combined.

Grease a large skillet with coconut oil and place it over medium-high heat.

Add the pancake batter in ½-cup measures, about 3 for a large skillet. Cook for about 3 minutes until the edges are firm, the bottom is golden, and the bubbles on the surface break. Flip and cook for about 2 minutes more until the other side is golden brown and the pancakes are cooked through. Transfer to a plate and wipe the skillet with a clean paper towel.

Re-grease the skillet and repeat until the remaining batter is used.

Serve the pancakes warm with fresh fruit, if desired.

Nutrition:

Calories: 286;

Total Fat: 17g;

Saturated Fat: 12g;

Carbohydrates: 27g;

Fiber: 1g;

Protein: 6g

Artichoke Frittata

Difficulty Level: 2/5

Preparation time: 10 minutes

Cooking time: 15 minutes

Servings: 4

Ingredients:

8 large eggs

¼ cup grated Asiago cheese

1 tablespoon chopped fresh basil

1 teaspoon chopped fresh oregano

Pinch sea salt

Pinch freshly ground black pepper

1 teaspoon extra-virgin olive oil

1 teaspoon minced garlic

1 cup canned, water-packed, quartered artichoke hearts, drained

1 tomato, chopped

Directions:

Preheat the oven to broil.

In a medium bowl, whisk the eggs, Asiago cheese, basil, oregano, sea salt, and pepper to blend.

Place a large ovenproof skillet over medium-high heat and add the olive oil. Add the garlic and sauté for 1 minute.

Remove the skillet from the heat and pour in the egg mixture.

Return the skillet to the heat and evenly sprinkle the artichoke hearts and tomato over the eggs.

Cook the frittata without stirring for about 8 minutes, or until the center is set.

Place the skillet under the broiler for about 1 minute, or until the top is lightly browned and puffed.

Cut the frittata into 4 pieces and serve.

Nutrition:

Calories: 199;

Total Fat: 13g;

Saturated Fat: 5g;

Carbohydrates: 5g;

Fiber: 2g;

Protein: 16g

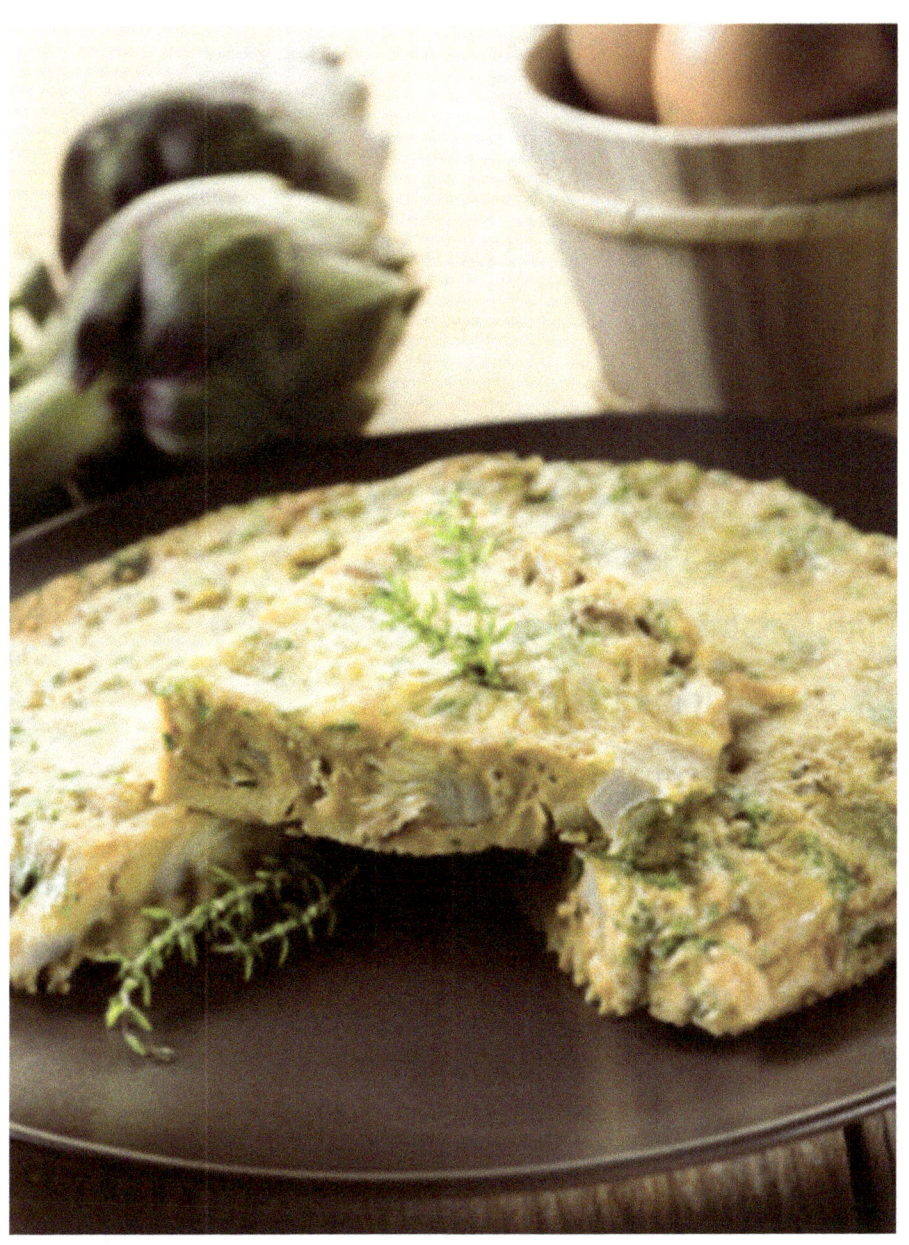

Fennel Wild Rice

Difficulty Level: 2/5

Preparation time: 10 minutes

Cooking time: 11 minutes

Servings: 6

Ingredients:

1 tablespoon extra-virgin olive oil

1 cup diced fennel

½ red bell pepper, finely diced

½ cup chopped sweet onion

2 cups cooked wild rice

1 tablespoon chopped fresh parsley

Sea salt

Freshly ground black pepper

Directions:

In a large skillet over medium-high heat, heat the olive oil.

Add the fennel, red bell pepper, and onion. Sauté for about 6 minutes, or until tender.

Stir in the wild rice. Cook for about 5 minutes until heated through.

Add the parsley, and season with sea salt and pepper.

Nutrition:

Calories: 222;

Total Fat: 3g;

Saturated Fat: 0g;

Carbohydrates: 43g;

Fiber: 4g;

Protein: 8g

Brussels Sprouts with Pistachios

Difficulty Level: 2/5

Preparation time: 15 minutes

Cooking time: 15 minutes

Servings: 4

Ingredients:

1 pound Brussels sprouts, tough bottoms trimmed, halved lengthwise

4 shallots, peeled and quartered

1 tablespoon extra-virgin olive oil

Sea salt

Freshly ground black pepper

½ cup chopped roasted pistachios

Zest of ½ lemon

Juice of ½ lemon

Directions:

Preheat the oven to 400°F.

Line a baking sheet with aluminum foil and set aside.

In a large bowl, toss the Brussels sprouts and shallots with the olive oil until well coated.

Season with sea salt and pepper, and then spread the vegetables evenly on the sheet.

Bake for 15 minutes, or until tender and lightly caramelized.

Remove from the oven and transfer to a serving bowl.

Toss with the pistachios, lemon zest, and lemon juice. Serve warm.

Nutrition:

Calories: 126;

Total Fat: 7g;

Saturated Fat: 1g;

Carbohydrates: 14g;

Fiber: 5g;

Protein: 6g

Roasted Parmesan Broccoli

Difficulty Level: 2/5

Preparation time: 10 minutes

Cooking time: 10 minutes

Servings: 4

Ingredients:

2 heads broccoli, cut into small florets

2 tablespoons extra-virgin olive oil, plus more for greasing the baking sheet

2 teaspoons minced garlic

Zest of 1 lemon

Juice of 1 lemon

Pinch sea salt

½ cup grated Parmesan cheese

Directions:

Preheat the oven to 400°F.

Lightly grease a baking sheet with olive oil and set aside.

In a large bowl, toss the broccoli with the 2 tablespoons of olive oil, garlic, lemon zest, lemon juice, and sea salt

Spread the mixture on the baking sheet in a single layer and sprinkle with the Parmesan cheese.

Bake for about 10 minutes, or until tender. Transfer the broccoli to a serving dish and serve.

Nutrition:

Calories: 154;

Total Fat: 11g;

Saturated Fat: 3g;

Carbohydrates: 10g;

Fiber: 4;

Protein: 9g

Mashed Celeriac

Difficulty Level: 2/5

Preparation time: 10 minutes

Cooking time: 20 minutes

Servings: 4

Ingredients:

2 celeriac (celery root), washed, peeled, and diced

2 teaspoons extra-virgin olive oil

1 tablespoon honey

½ teaspoon ground nutmeg

Sea salt

Freshly ground black pepper

Directions:

Preheat the oven to 400°F.

Line a baking sheet with aluminum foil and set aside.

In a large bowl, toss together the celeriac and olive oil. Spread the celeriac pieces evenly on the baking sheet, and roast for about 20 minutes until very tender and lightly caramelized. Transfer to a large bowl.

Add the honey and nutmeg. Use a potato masher to mash the ingredients until fluffy.

Season with sea salt and pepper before serving.

Nutrition:

Calories: 136;

Total Fat: 3g;

Saturated Fat: 1g;

Carbohydrates: 26g;

Fiber: 4g;

Protein: 4g

Herbed Yogurt Dip

Difficulty Level: 1/5

Preparation time: 10 minutes

Cooking time: 0 minutes

Servings: 4

Ingredients:

1 cup plain Greek yogurt

Zest of ½ lemon

Juice of ½ lemon

1 tablespoon finely chopped fresh chives

2 teaspoons chopped fresh dill

2 teaspoons chopped fresh thyme

1 teaspoon chopped fresh parsley

½ teaspoon minced garlic

Pinch sea salt

Directions:

In a medium bowl, stir together the yogurt, lemon zest, lemon juice, chives, dill, thyme, parsley, and garlic until very well blended.

Season with the sea salt and transfer to a sealed container.

Keep refrigerated for up to 2 weeks.

Nutrition:

Calories: 59;

Total Fat: 4g;

Saturated Fat: 2g;

Carbohydrates: 5g;

Fiber: 4g;

Protein: 2g

Southwest Pizza

Difficulty Level: 2/5

Preparation time: 15 minutes

Cooking time: 10 minutes

Servings: 4

Ingredients:

4 (6-inch) whole-wheat pita breads

1 tablespoon extra-virgin olive oil

2 cups canned sodium-free white navy beans, drained and rinsed

1 scallion, white and green parts, finely chopped

1 jalapeño pepper, seeded and finely chopped

1 teaspoon ground cumin

1 tomato, diced

1 yellow bell pepper, thinly sliced

½ cup crumbled feta cheese

4 teaspoons chopped fresh cilantro

Directions:

Preheat the oven to 400°F.

Place the pita breads on a baking sheet and lightly brush both sides with olive oil. Bake for about 5 minutes until golden brown and crispy, turning once.

In a medium bowl, mash together the beans, scallion, jalapeño, and cumin to form a chunky paste.

Evenly divide the bean mixture among the toasted pita breads, spreading it to the edges.

Top each with tomato, yellow bell pepper, and feta cheese.

Bake the pizzas for about 3 minutes until the cheese is slightly melted.

Sprinkle with cilantro and serve.

Nutrition:

Calories: 387;

Total Fat: 9g;

Saturated Fat: 3g;

Carbohydrates: 64g;

Fiber: 16g;

Protein: 17g

Spinach Chicken Pizza

Difficulty Level: 2/5

Preparation time: 15 minutes

Cooking time: 15 minutes

Servings: 4

Ingredients:

1 (9-inch) pizza crust, homemade or premade

½ teaspoon extra-virgin olive oil

1 cup chopped tomato

¼ teaspoon red pepper flakes

2 cups chopped blanched fresh spinach

1 tablespoon chopped fresh basil

1 cup chopped cooked chicken breast

1 cup shredded Asiago cheese

Directions:

Preheat the oven to 400°F.

Prepare the pizza dough according to your recipe or package instructions and roll it out to form a 9-inch crust. Transfer the crust to a baking sheet, and brush the edges lightly with olive oil.

Spread the tomato and red pepper flakes over the pizza leaving the oiled crust bare.

Arrange the spinach and basil over the tomato, and scatter the chopped chicken on the spinach. Top with the Asiago cheese.

Bake the pizza for about 15 minutes until the crust is crispy and the cheese is melted.

Nutrition:

Calories: 255;

Total Fat: 11g;

Saturated Fat: 5g;

Carbohydrates: 17g;

Fiber: 2g;

Protein: 23g

Linguine with Cherry Tomatoes

Difficulty Level: 2/5

Preparation time: 10 minutes

Cooking time: 15 minutes

Servings: 4

Ingredients:

2 pounds cherry tomatoes

3 tablespoons extra-virgin olive oil

2 tablespoons balsamic vinegar

2 teaspoons minced garlic

Pinch freshly ground black pepper

¾ pound whole-wheat linguine pasta

1 tablespoon chopped fresh oregano

¼ cup crumbled feta cheese

Directions:

Preheat the oven to 350°F.

Line a baking sheet with parchment paper and set aside.

In a large bowl, toss the cherry tomatoes with 2 tablespoons of olive oil, the balsamic vinegar, garlic, and pepper until well coated. Spread the tomatoes evenly on the prepared sheet and roast for about 15 minutes until they are softened and burst open.

While the tomatoes roast, cook the pasta according to package directions. Drain and transfer to a large bowl.

Toss the pasta with the remaining 1 tablespoon of olive oil.

Add the roasted tomatoes, taking care to get all the juices and bits from the baking sheet. Toss to combine.

To serve, top with the oregano and feta cheese.

Nutrition:

Calories: 397;

Total Fat: 15g;

Saturated Fat: 3g;

Carbohydrates: 55g;

Fiber: 6g;

Protein: 13g

Linguine with Tomato Clam Sauce

Difficulty Level: 2/5

Preparation time: 10 minutes

Cooking time: 10minutes

Servings: 4

Ingredients:

1 pound linguine

Pinch sea salt

1 teaspoon extra-virgin olive oil

1 tablespoon minced garlic

1 teaspoon chopped fresh thyme

½ teaspoon red pepper flakes

1 (15-ounce) can sodium-free diced tomatoes, drained

1 (15-ounce) can whole baby clams, with their juice

Sea salt

Freshly ground black pepper

2 tablespoons chopped fresh parsley

Directions:

Cook the linguine according to the package directions.

While the linguine cooks, heat the olive oil in a large skillet over medium heat.

the garlic, thyme, and red pepper flakes. Sauté for about 3 minutes until softened.

Stir in the tomatoes and clams. Bring the sauce to a boil, reduce the heat to low, and simmer for 5 minutes.

Season with sea salt and pepper.

Drain the cooked pasta and toss it with the sauce.

Garnish with the parsley and serve.

Nutrition:

Calories: 394;

Total Fat: 5g;

Saturated Fat: 0g;

Carbohydrates: 66g;

Fiber: 7g;

Protein: 23g

Angel Hair with Asparagus-Kale Pesto

Difficulty Level: 2/5

Preparation time: 10 minutes

Cooking time: 10 minutes

Servings: 6

Ingredients:

¾ pound asparagus, woody ends removed, and coarsely chopped

¼ pound kale, thoroughly washed

½ cup grated Asiago cheese

¼ cup fresh basil

¼ cup extra-virgin olive oil

Juice of 1 lemon

Sea salt

Freshly ground black pepper

1 pound angel hair pasta

Zest of 1 lemon

Directions:

In a food processor, pulse the asparagus and kale until very finely chopped.

Add the Asiago cheese, basil, olive oil, and lemon juice and pulse to form a smooth pesto.

Season with sea salt and pepper and set aside.

Cook the pasta al dente according to the package directions. Drain and transfer to a large bowl.

Add the pesto, tossing well to coat.

Sprinkle with lemon zest and serve.

Nutrition:

Calories: 283;

Total Fat: 12g;

Saturated Fat: 2g;

Carbohydrates: 33g;

Fiber: 2g;

Protein: 10g

Cucumber Hummus Sandwiches

Difficulty Level: 1/5

Preparation time: 5 minutes

Cooking time: 0 minutes

Servings: 1

Ingredients:

10 round slices cucumber

5 teaspoons hummus

Instructions:

Add 1 teaspoon hummus on one slice of cucumber. Top with another slice and serve.

Nutritional info (per serving):

54 calories;

2.1 g fat;

7 g total carbs;

2 g protein

Blackberries Caprese Skewers

Difficulty Level: 2/5

Preparation time: 15 minutes

Cooking time: 0 minutes

Servings: 4

Ingredients:

½ cup cherry tomatoes

4 fresh basil leaves

4 blackberries

¼ cup baby mozzarella balls

Directions:

Put blackberries, tomatoes, mozzarella balls, and basil on skewers.

Once done, serve.

Nutritional info (per serving):

40 calories;

1.7 g fat;

4 g total carbs;

2 g protein

Tomato-Basil Skewers

Difficulty Level: 1/5

Preparation time: 15 minutes

Cooking time: 0 minutes

Servings: 6

Ingredients:

16 cherry tomatoes

16 fresh basil leaves

16 small fresh mozzarella balls

olive oil

salt and black pepper

Instructions:

Put mozzarella, basil, and tomatoes on skewers.

Add the oil and season well.

Once done, serve.

Nutritional info (per serving):

46 calories;

3.3 g fat;

1 g total carbs;

2.8 g protein

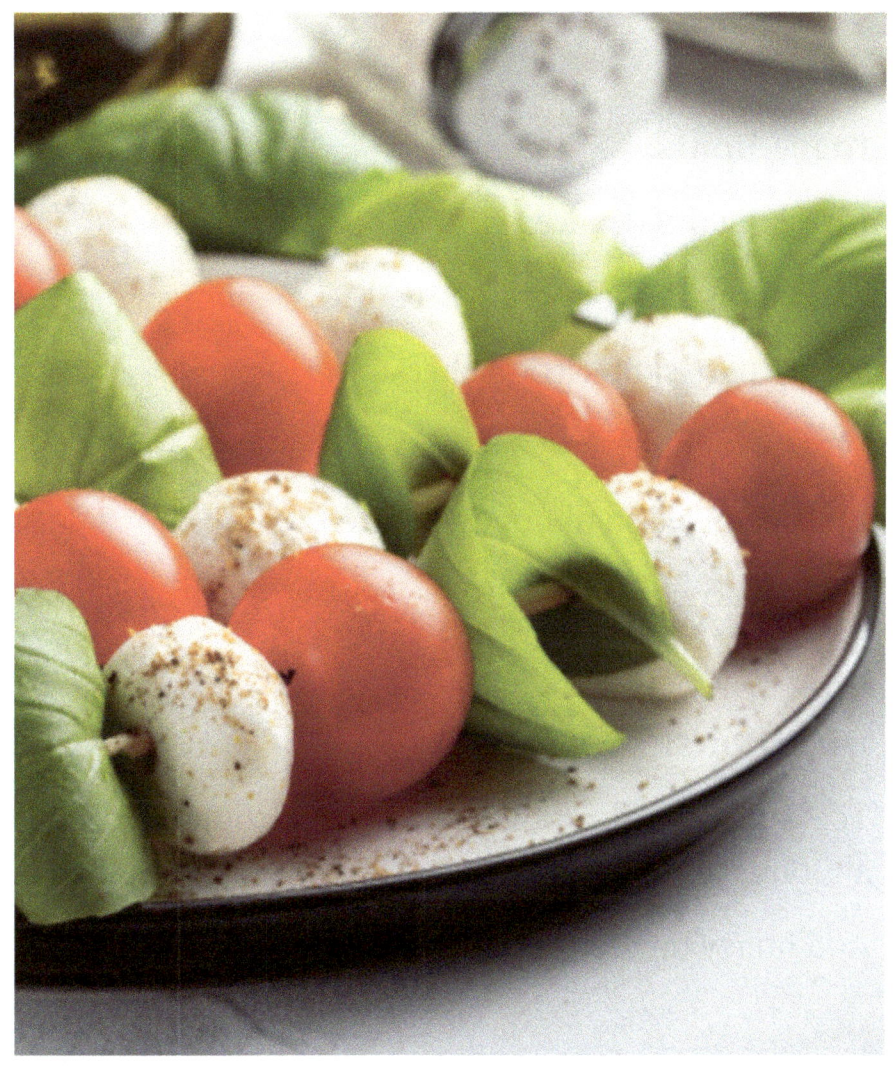

Fig and Ricotta Toast

Difficulty Level: 2/5

Preparation time: 10 minutes

Cooking time: 0 minutes

Servings: 1

Ingredients:

1 fresh fig dried, sliced

1 slice crusty whole-grain bread

¼ cup part-skim ricotta cheese

1 teaspoon honey

1 teaspoon sliced almonds, toasted

pinch flaky sea salt

Directions:

Toast the bread and add the figs, ricotta cheese, and almonds on it.

Add honey on top, season with sea salt, and serve.

Nutritional info (per serving):

252 calories;

9.1 g fat;

32.1 g total carbs;

12.5 g protein

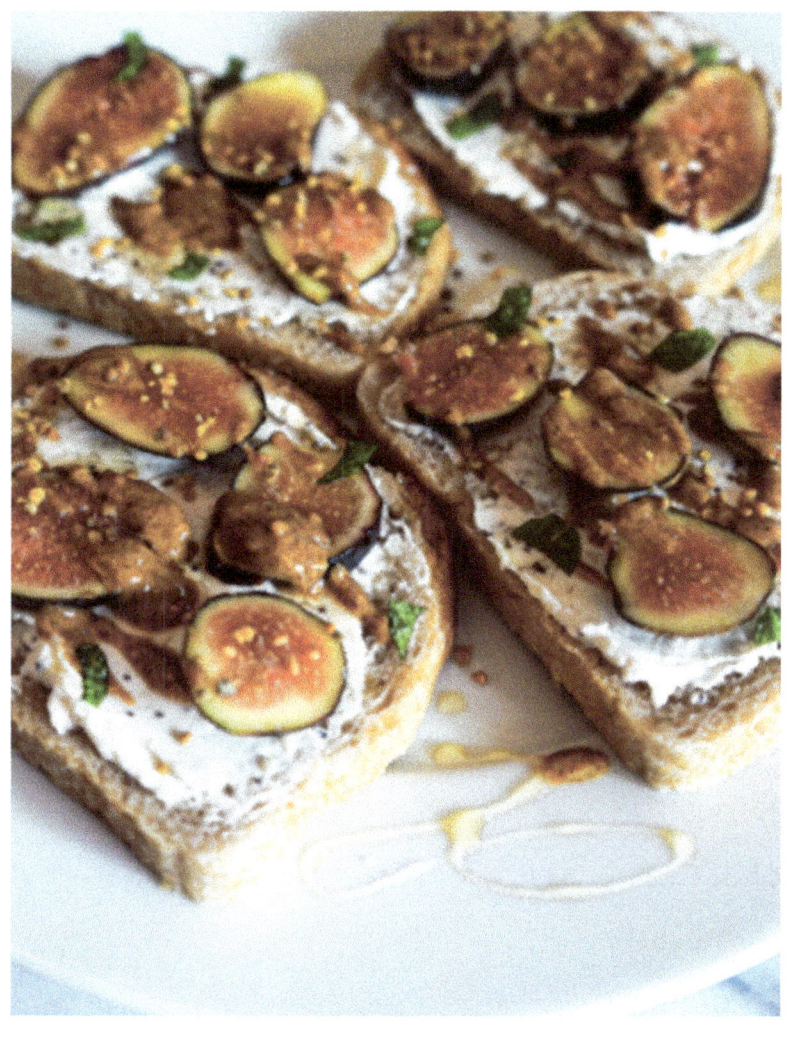

Date Wraps

Difficulty Level: 1/5
Preparation time: 10 minutes
Cooking time: 0 minutes
Servings: 16 bites

Ingredients:

16 whole pitted dates

16 thin slices prosciutto

pepper

Directions:

Place prosciutto slice flat on a plate. Put a date into it and wrap the slice around it.

Repeat with the remaining, season with pepper and serve.

Nutritional info (per serving):

35 calories;

0.8 g fat;

5.6 g total carbs;

2.2 g protein

Easy Stuffed Peppers

Difficulty Level: 2/5

Preparation time: 5 minutes

Cooking time: 10 minutes

Servings: 4

Ingredients:

2 tablespoon pesto sauce

4 red peppers

1 lb. cooked tomato rice

2 cups goat cheese, sliced

handful black olives, pitted

Directions:

Cut the top of the red peppers and scoop out the seeds. Place the peppers on the plate, cut side up, and microwave for 6 minutes on high.

Mix the rice with pesto with a handful of black olives, and 1 3/8 cup cheese. Add this mixture on the peppers and top with the remaining cheese. Cook for 10 minutes.

Serve.

Nutritional info (per serving):

387 calories;

17 g fat;

46 g total carbs;

15 g protein

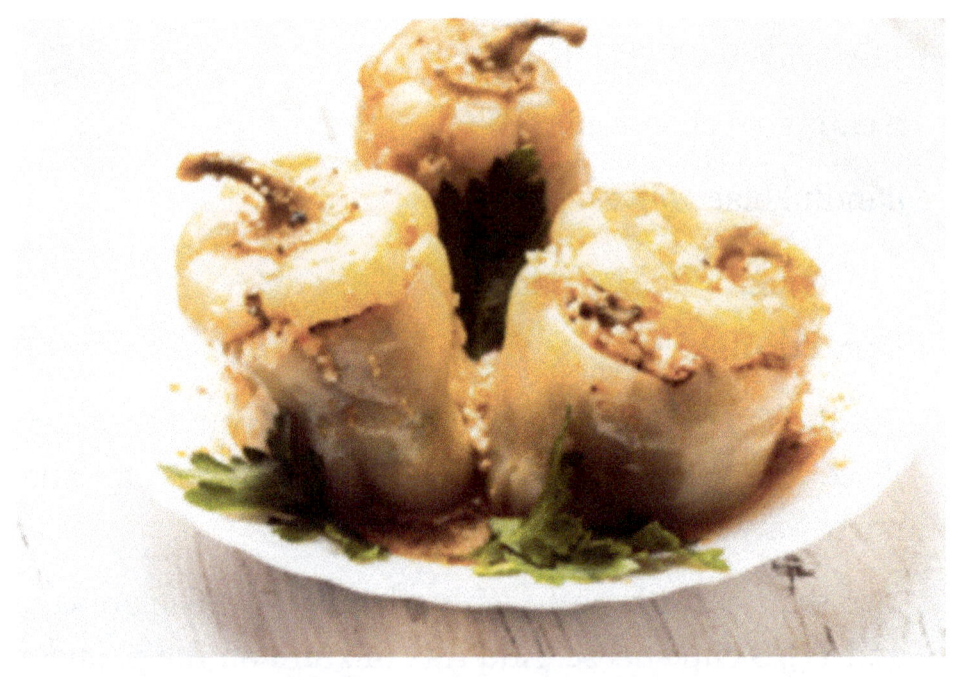

Buttery Carrot Sticks

Difficulty Level: 2/5

Preparation time: 10 minutes

Cooking time: 15 minutes

Serves: 4

Ingredients:

1 pound carrot, cut into sticks

4 garlic cloves, minced

¼ cup chicken stock

1 teaspoon rosemary, chopped

A pinch of salt and black pepper

2 tablespoons olive oil

2 tablespoons ghee, melted

Directions:

Set the pressure pot on Sauté mode, add the oil and the ghee, heat them up, add the garlic and brown for 1 minute.

Add the rest of the ingredients, put the lid on and cook on High for 14 minutes.

Release the pressure naturally for 10 minutes, arrange the carrot sticks on a platter and serve.

Nutrition:

Calories 142,

Fat 4g,

Fiber 2g,

Carbohydrates 5g,

Protein 7g

Cajun Walnuts and Olives Bowls

Difficulty Level: 2/5

Preparation time: 10 minutes

Cooking time: 10 minutes

Serves: 2

Ingredients:

½ pound walnuts, chopped

A pinch of salt and black pepper

1 and ½ cups black olives, pitted

½ tablespoon Cajun seasoning

2 garlic cloves, minced

1 red chili pepper, chopped

¼ cup veggie stock

2 tablespoon tomato puree

Directions:

In your pressure pot, combine the walnuts with the olives and the rest of the ingredients, put the lid on and cook on High 10 minutes.

Release the pressure fast for 5 minutes, divide the mix into small bowls and serve as an appetizer.

Nutrition:

Calories 105,

Fat 1g,

Fiber 1g,

Carbohydrates 4g,

Protein 7g

Mango Salsa

Difficulty Level: 2/5

Preparation time: 10 minutes

Cooking time: 10 minutes

Serves: 2

Ingredients:

2 mangoes, peeled and cubed

½ tablespoon sweet paprika

2 garlic cloves, minced

2 tablespoons cilantro, chopped

1 tablespoon spring onions, chopped

1 cup cherry tomatoes, cubed

1 cup avocado, peeled, pitted and cubed

A pinch of salt and black pepper

1 tablespoon olive oil

¼ cup tomato puree

½ cup kalamata olives, pitted and sliced

Directions:

In your pressure pot, combine the mangoes with the paprika and the rest of the ingredients except the cilantro, put the lid on and cook on High for 5 minutes.

Release the pressure fast for 5 minutes, divide the mix into small bowls, sprinkle the cilantro on top and serve.

Nutrition:

Calories 123,

Fat 4g,

Fiber 1g,

Carbs 3g,

Protein 5g

Crisp Spiced Cauliflower with Feta Cheese

Difficulty Level: 2/5

Preparation time: 5 minutes

Cooking time: 10 minutes

Serves: 4

Ingredients:

3/4 lb cauliflower, chopped

1/2 Tbsp. ground toasted cumin seeds

1 garlic clove, grated

2 Tbsp. crumbled feta cheese

1 1/2 Tbsp. freshly squeezed lemon juice

1 Tbsp. chopped fresh flat leaf parsley

Chili flakes

Sweet smoked paprika

Sea salt

Canola oil

Directions:

Place a skillet over high flame and heat just enough canola oil to cover the bottom.

Allow the oil to smoke slightly, then add the chopped cauliflower and stir fry for about 2 minutes or until browned and crisp. Season with salt.

Reduce to medium flame as you continue to stir fry the cauliflower. Sprinkle in the cumin, lemon juice, grated garlic, and a dash of chili flakes, then stir well to combine.

Transfer the cauliflower to a platter, then top with feta, parsley, and a dash of paprika. Serve right away.

Nutrition:

Calories 300,

Fat 19.3 g,

Carbohydrates 30.6 g,

Sugar 8.8 g,

Protein 3.4 g,

Cholesterol 0 mg

Spring Peas and Beans with Zesty Thyme Yogurt Sauce

Difficulty Level: 3/5

Preparation time: 5 minutes

Cooking time: 10 minutes

Serves: 4

Ingredients:

3/4 lb fresh shelling beans, shelled

3/4 lb fresh peas (such as English peas, edamame, etc.), shelled

1 lb pole beans, preferably assorted (such as purple wax, Romano, and yellow)

6 young pea shoots

1/2 tsp. ground sumac

1 1/2 Tbsp. extra virgin olive oil

Sea salt

For the Zesty Thyme Yogurt Sauce:

1/4 cup Greek yogurt

1 1/2 Tbsp. fresh thyme leaves

1 garlic clove, grated

1/2 lemon, juiced and zested

Cayenne

Sea salt

Directions:

Combine all the ingredients for the yogurt sauce in a bowl, then season to taste with salt and cayenne. Cover the bowl and refrigerate until ready to serve.

Prepare a bowl of ice water and set aside.

Boil some salted water in a saucepan, then add the fresh beans and peas. Boil for 2 minutes, or until tender, then remove immediately with a metal mesh strainer and plunge into the ice water to prevent them from being soggy.

Blot the peas and beans dry using paper towels, then place in a large bowl and set aside.

Refill the bowl of ice water.

Boil the salted water in the saucepan again, then add the pole beans and cook for 2 minutes or until almost tender. Remove immediately with a metal mesh strainer and plunge into the ice water to prevent them from being soggy.

Blot the pole beans dry using paper towels, then add to the bowl of peas and beans. Toss everything to combine.

Drizzle the olive oil over the peas and beans, then season with salt and sumac. Toss well to combine, then add the yogurt sauce on top. Garnish with pea shoots and thyme, then serve right away.

Nutrition:

Calories 153,

Fat 0.5 g,

Carbohydrates 39.1 g,

Sugar 25.7 g,

Protein 1.2 g,

Cholesterol 0 mg

Breakfast Pita

Difficulty Level: 2/5

Preparation Time: 15 minutes

Cooking time: 15 minutes

Servings: 4

Ingredients:

4 pita breads

2 eggs, whisked

4 oz. ham, chopped

1 tablespoon olive oil

¼ teaspoon salt

4 oz. Parmesan, grated

1 cup water

Directions:

Rub the pitas with the olive oil. Place them in ramekins and put them on the trivet.

Combine the whisked eggs, ham, salt, and grated cheese in the mixing bowl.

Pour the egg mixture into the ramekins with pita and transfer the trivet into the pressure pot.

Pour the water into the bottom of the Pressure pot bowl.

Close the lid and cook the pitas for 15 minutes on High pressure.

Do a natural pressure release and serve the breakfast!

Nutrition:

Calories 199,

Fat 15.1,

Fiber 2,

Carbohydrates 45.4,

Protein 22.6

Beef with Pesto Sandwich

Difficulty Level: 2/5

Preparation time: 5 minutes

Cooking Time: 20 minutes

Servings: 4

Ingredients:

4 slices mozzarella cheese

½ lb. thinly sliced roast beef deli

¼ cup basil pesto

2 tbsp softened butter

8 slices, ½-inch thick Italian bread

Directions:

Spread the butter on one side of four of the bread slices, then top with pesto and evenly spread.

Top with beef, then cheese slices and cover with the un-buttered bread slice.

Place on a Panini pan and grill until crispy. Serve and enjoy.

Nutrition:

Calories per Serving: 248;

Carbohydrates: 2.5g;

Protein: 23.3g;

Fat: 15.8g

Classic Steak Panini

Difficulty Level: 2/5

Preparation time: 5 minutes

Cooking time: 12 minutes

Servings: 2

Ingredients:

2 tbsp yellow mustard

2 tbsp softened butter

1 baguette or ciabatta roll

Ground pepper and salt

2 thin slices of minute steaks

2 large onions peeled and sliced

2 tbsp olive oil

Directions:

On a heated skillet pour half of the oil and cook onions until browned and translucent, around ten minutes.

Season steak with salt and pepper. Then, gather thee onions on one end of the skillet and pour in the remaining oil as you pan fry the seasoned steak on high heat.

Cooking each side for at least 45 seconds and remove from fire and set aside.

Halve your bread lengthwise and arrange the steaks topped by onions and cover with the other bread half. Grill your sandwich in a Panini pan for at least 3 minutes.

Serve with your favorite condiment.

Nutrition:

Calories per Serving: 529;

Carbohydrates: 27.7g;

Protein: 14.0g;

Fat: 41.8g

Grilled Sandwich with Goat Cheese

Difficulty Level: 2/5

Preparation time: 10 minutes

Cooking time: 8 minutes

Servings: 4

Ingredients:

½ cup soft goat cheese

4 Kaiser rolls 2-oz

¼ tsp freshly ground black pepper

¼ tsp salt

1/3 cup chopped basil

Cooking spray

4 big Portobello mushroom caps

1 yellow bell pepper, cut in half and seeded

1 red bell pepper, cut in half and seeded

1 garlic clove, minced

1 tbsp olive oil

¼ cup balsamic vinegar

Directions:

In a large bowl, mix garlic, olive oil and balsamic vinegar. Add mushroom and bell peppers. Gently mix to coat. Remove veggies from vinegar and discard vinegar mixture.

Coat with cooking spray a grill rack and the grill preheated to medium high fire.

Place mushrooms and bell peppers on the grill and grill for 4 minutes per side. Remove from grill and let cool a bit.

Into thin strips, cut the bell peppers.

In a small bowl, combine black pepper, salt, basil and sliced bell peppers.

Horizontally, cut the Kaiser rolls and evenly spread cheese on the cut side.

Arrange 1 Portobello per roll, top with 1/3 bell pepper mixture and cover with the other half of the roll.

Grill the rolls as you press down on them to create a Panini like line on the bread. Grill until bread is toasted.

Nutrition:

Calories per Serving: 317;

Carbohydrates: 41.7g;

Protein: 14.0g;

Fat: 10.5g

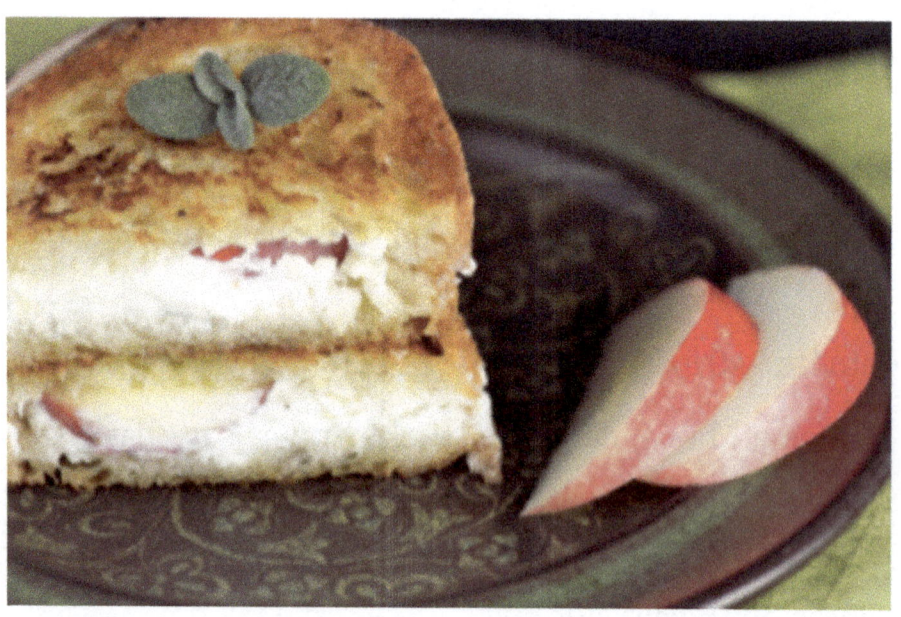

Fried Green Tomatoes

Difficulty Level: 2/5

Preparation time: 10 minutes

Cooking time: 8 minutes

Servings: 4

Ingredients

1 tablespoon Vegetable Oil

½ teaspoon Black Pepper

½ teaspoon Salt

½ cup Bread Crumbs

½ cup Cornmeal

1 cup All-purpose Flour

½ cup Milk

2 Eggs

4 Green Tomatoes

Directions

Pour the vegetable oil into a large pan and begin to heat it up into a medium heat.

While the oil heats, you will want to prepare your tomatoes by slicing them into half inch thick pieces.

Be sure to throw the ends out as you will have no need for them. In a bowl, mix together the milk and the eggs.

Place your flour onto a plate and line up with the bowl that is holding the milk and eggs.

On a third plate, mix together your breadcrumbs, cornmeal, pepper, and salt.

Now that these are prepared, dip your tomato pieces in the liquid mixture, the flour, and then the breadcrumb mixture. Be sure to coat the tomatoes before tossing them into the vegetable oil.

Fry the tomatoes for five minutes on either side or until golden brown. Portion them out and enjoy as a side dish or a nice, healthy snack!

Nutrition:

Calories per Serving: 298;

Carbs: 61.1g;

Protein: 7.4g;

Fat: 5.0g

One-of-a-Kind Veggie Slaw

Difficulty Level: 2/5

Preparation time: 10 minutes

Cooking time: 20 minutes

Servings: 6

Ingredients:

2 tsp salt

2 tbsp Bavarian seasoning

½ cup lightly packed fresh mint leaves

½ cup fresh lemon juice

½ cup roasted and shelled pistachios, roughly chopped

6 oz dried cranberries

4 bacon strips, cooked to a crisp (keep rendered fat) and chopped to bits

1/3 cup extra virgin olive oil (use rendered fat from bacon to reach ½ cup)

2 lbs. Brussels sprouts, cleaned and trimmed of large stem pieces

Directions:

Shred Brussels sprouts in a food processor. Transfer into a large salad bowl.

In a small bowl mix salt, Bavarian seasoning, mint and lemon juice.

Then slowly add oil while whisking continuously and vigorously. Add more seasoning to taste if needed.

Pour half of dressing into the salad bowl, toss to mix and add more if needed.

Top salad with bacon pieces, dried cranberries and pistachios before serving.

Nutrition:

Calories per Serving: 343.8;

Carbohydrates: 38.7g;

Protein: 9.7g;

Fat: 20.0g

Ratatouille Grilled Style

Difficulty Level: 2/5

Preparation time:

Cooking time: 20 minutes

Servings: 4

Ingredients:

2 tbsp walnuts, toasted and chopped

2 tbsp apple cider

2 tbsp extra virgin olive oil

2 medium yellow squash, cut into ¼" rounds

1 large zucchini, cut into ¼" rounds

1 large zucchini, cut into ¼" rounds

1 large Portobello mushroom cap, cut into ¼" slices

1 medium eggplant, cut into ¼" rounds

1 red bell pepper, quartered, stems and seeds removed

1 large red onion, cut into ¼" slices

Directions:

Preheat grill to medium high and lightly grease grill pan with cooking spray.

Place all sliced veggies in grill pan and drizzle with olive oil. Toss well to coat.

Place in grill and grill for ten minutes. Toss vegetables to ensure even heating and continue grilling for another 10 minutes.

Toss vegetables and check if lightly charred and cooked through. If needed, grill some more to desired doneness.

Transfer grilled veggies into salad bowl, add walnuts and zero belly dressing. T

Toss to combine well, serve and enjoy.

Nutrition:

Calories per Serving: 212;

Carbs: 27.6g;

Protein: 7.4g;

Fat: 10.6g

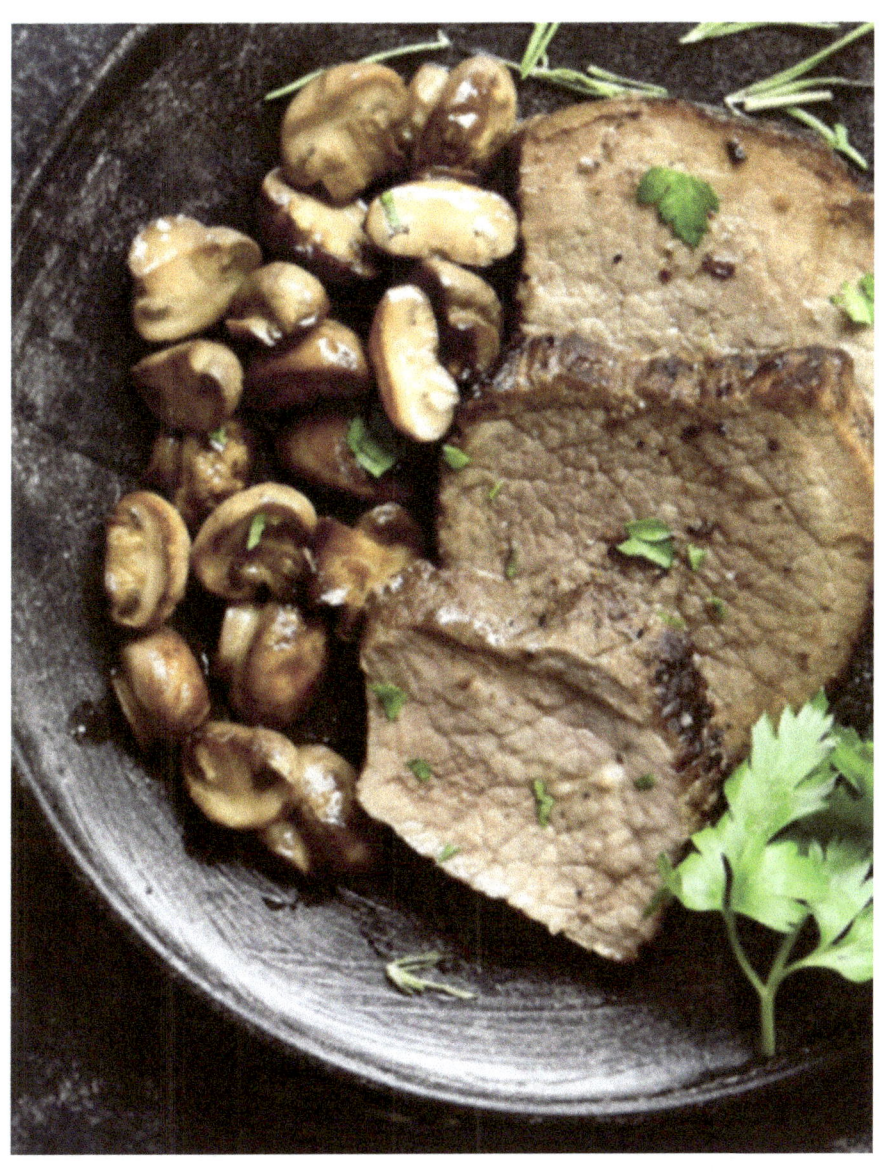

Lightning Source UK Ltd.
Milton Keynes UK
UKHW020721270521
384465UK00005B/128